BREATHING
THROUGH THE
WHOLE BODY

"I love every word! Thank you so much for bringing forth such a succinct and glowingly accurate account of the central role that body wisdom, somatic experiencing, plays in the process of awakening. It is a 'how to do it' book for all of us on this road to realizing our true nature."

ROBERT HALL, BUDDHIST TEACHER AND
COFOUNDER OF THE LOMI SCHOOL

Breathing
THROUGH THE
Whole Body

The Buddha's Instructions
on Integrating
Mind, Body, and Breath

WILL JOHNSON

Inner Traditions
Rochester, Vermont • Toronto, Canada

Inner Traditions
One Park Street
Rochester, Vermont 05767
www.InnerTraditions.com

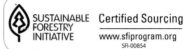

SUSTAINABLE FORESTRY INITIATIVE
Certified Sourcing
www.sfiprogram.org
SFI-00854

Text stock is SFI certified

Library of Congress Cataloging-in-Publication Data
Johnson, Will, 1946–
  Breathing through the whole body : the Buddha's instructions on
integrating mind, body, and breath / Will Johnson.
    p. cm.
  Includes index.
  Summary: "Explores the Buddha's own words on breathing meditation
for healing, wholeness, and a deeper understanding of his teachings"—
Provided by publisher.
  ISBN 978-1-59477-434-8 (pbk.) — ISBN 978-1-59477-710-3 (e-book)
  1. Anapanasmrti. 2. Gautama Buddha—Quotations. I. Title.
  BQ5630.A6J65 2012
  294.3'4446—dc23
                                                    2011040119

Printed and bound in the United States by Lake Book Manufacturing
The text stock is SFI certified. The Sustainable Forestry Initiative®
program promotes sustainable forest management.

10 9 8 7 6 5 4 3 2 1

Text design and layout by Virginia Scott Bowman
This book was typeset in Garamond Premier Pro, Gentle Sans, and
Cochin with Trajan Pro and Trade Gothic used as display typefaces

To send correspondence to the author of this book, mail a first-class
letter to the author c/o Inner Traditions • Bear & Company, One Park
Street, Rochester, VT 05767, and we will forward the communication,
or contact the author directly at **www.embodiment.net**.

To Asclepiades

As always, the good folks at Inner Traditions have been extremely helpful and supportive in shepherding this little book from my computer to your hands and eyes. Over the years, they've become friends as much as professional contributors. Special thanks go to Jamaica Burns Griffin, Jon Graham, Jeanie Levitan, and Nancy Yeilding.

PART TWO

THE BREATH OF
UNENDING MOTION

CONTENTS

. . . FROM *THE SATIPATTHANA SUTTA*

go to a quiet place in the wilderness,
the forest,
or even a room in an empty building

sitting down in a posture of meditation,
keeping the spine upright and erect,
begin by observing the breath in the front of the body

remain aware as you breathe in
remain aware as you breathe out

notice if the breath is long or short

as you breathe in, breathe in through the whole body
as you breathe out, breathe out through the whole body

feel how the breath calms and heals the body

like a skilled potter watching clay turn on a wheel
notice how each inhalation turns into an exhalation
only to turn back again into an inhalation
over and over and over again

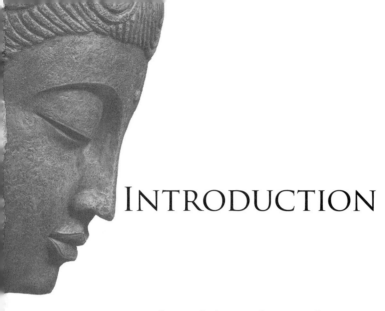

INTRODUCTION

From our very first inhalation that signals entrance into the world to our very last exhalation through which we bid the world a final farewell, breath is with us our entire life. It is our constant and most reliable companion (our heart may skip a beat from time to time, but we never miss a breath), never abandoning us or leaving our side. It provides us—moment by moment, breath by breath—with the most vital nourishment we need to keep our body alive. Take food away from us, and we can live for several months. Take water away from us, and we can survive for several days. Cut off the life-sustaining oxygen in the air we breathe for even a few minutes, and our body dies. Breathing in . . . breathing out . . .

So vital to our survival is the action of breathing that, much like the systolic and diastolic beating of our heart, its rhythmic repetitions of inhalation and exhalation keep occurring whether or not we're aware of them. While we have no choice but to breathe, we have the ability to affect how we breathe. We can slow the breath down. We can speed it up. We can cause it to become fuller or slighter, stronger or weaker. We

1

can consciously yield to its primal impulse and rhythms, or we can unconsciously constrain it and hold back its force.

Breath can flow freely, like a stream in spring, or it can become stagnant, its current jammed. Chronic tensions in the body and contractions in the mind interfere with the free flow of breath. Like logjams in a river, they can slow breath down to a trickle. Surrendering to breath's current brings more vibrancy to the body and peace to the mind. Bracing against its current keeps the body sluggish and the mind overactive. Either pattern can keep the body alive, but only one keeps the body happy.

Because restrictions to breath can be eased and altered, and because this alteration can so dramatically affect not only the vibrancy of the body but the condition of the mind itself, spiritual teachers—from times too ancient to have been recorded right up to the present day—have relied on different techniques and practices of breathing to help students gain insight. Many of the techniques are energizing, others deeply relaxing. Some mold the breath, forming it into specific shapes and patterns; others just watch it, accepting it exactly as it is. All of them connect us with our body. The common denominator of the many different traditions and schools of Buddhism, each with their own unique approach to practice, is their shared interest in the breath. Starting 2,500 years ago with the seminal teachings of the historical Buddha, the Indian prince Siddhartha Gotama, and moving through every intervening century since, Buddhist teachers from all traditions have been telling us, in one form or another, to breathe and be aware.

The three historical *suttas* (or texts) that speak of the breath most prominently, and whose statements have been directly attributed to the Buddha himself, are the *Satipatthana Sutta,* the *Anapanasati Sutta,* and the *Kayagatasati Sutta.* Here can be found the Buddha's actual instructions on meditation, and these instructions are as germane today as when they were first uttered 2,500 years ago. All three of these texts include specific instructions about breath, and the breath practices in many of our contemporary Buddhist schools are still based on interpretations of the words in these texts.

The principal instructions on meditating on the breath in all three of these suttas are fundamentally identical. The meditator is encouraged to go to a quiet place where he or she won't be too disturbed or distracted, sit down in such a way that the spine remains erect, and begin to observe the passage of breath at the front of the body. The two most common contemporary interpretations of the opening instructions in these suttas tell the meditator to keep his or her mind completely focused and concentrated on the action of the breath as it can be observed and felt in one of two very specific, isolated spots, both at the front of the body: the area of the nostrils (where one can observe and feel the breath as it enters and leaves the body) or the abdomen (where one can pay attention to how the action of breath causes the belly to rise and fall, expand and contract, on every inhalation and exhalation).

Through this kind of focused attention, mind stays more tethered to the present moment. Breathing in . . . breathing out . . . Indeed, one of the primary purposes of the practice is to calm the tendency of the mind to jump around from thought to thought so it can remain more present and aware. Thoughts in the mind are almost entirely either reminiscences about the past or projections into the future, and—as Buddhist teachers are fond of pointing out—the past and the future have no existential reality other than as thoughts in the present moment. Only the experience of this moment has a claim to being real (it is certainly the only moment that is directly *experienceable*), and the Buddha discovered that grounding our awareness in the ever-changing reality of the present moment keeps us from getting tangled up in thought realms that all too easily lead to distortions of perception.

Curiously, however, there is another statement about the breath in all three of these suttas that is often overlooked in most contemporary Buddhist schools. Instead of just observing the breath as it acts on one small, isolated part of the body, the Buddha also quite clearly encouraged his students to do the following:

as you breathe in, breathe in through the whole body
as you breathe out, breathe out through the whole body

While this passage hasn't found its way into practice anywhere nearly so prevalently as the more isolating instruction to observe the activity of breath in one specific part of the body to the exclusion of all others, it has been the subject of much debate among Buddhist scholars and teachers. While some scholars insist that the passage refers to the *whole body of the breath*—the taking in of the breath, the filling up of the lungs, and the expelling out of the breath—others suggest that, no, it really is referring to the physical body itself and to some kind of merging of body with breath.

It is my view that the latter interpretation is much closer to what the Buddha originally intended, and it is this view on which the explanation of this passage in this book is based.

In this, I'm supported by the contemporary Buddhist scholar-practitioner Thanissaro Bhikkhu who, in commenting on this passage from the suttas, says: "the step of breathing in and out sensitive to the entire body relates to the many similes in the suttas depicting *jhana* [a deep absorption in the essence of the mind] as a state of whole-body awareness."*

I would also hasten to add that, in actual practice, there's little difference between either of these interpretations for, as we will see, it is not possible to breathe through the entire length of the breath without also feeling how that breath stimulates the whole of the body. Nor is it possible to experience the entire tactile field of the body (the state of whole-body awareness about which Thanissaro Bhikkhu speaks) without also surrendering to a full and complete breath.

Keeping our entire attention focused on one small part of the body can significantly help develop our powers of concentration (what the Buddha referred to as *samadhi*), and there are very real benefits that come from developing strong concentration. Concentration alone, however, has never been presented as the final goal of Buddhist practice. It is a very important stepping-stone on the path, a necessary skill that allows the practitioner to move more easily and gracefully into the unusual terrain of *panna* (or wisdom) where the mind doesn't just remain concentrated but is actually able to confront its essence nakedly, directly, and boldly. To enter the field of panna, the practitioner will want to open himself or herself to everything that can be experienced, not just one isolated aspect of it: the

---

*From Thanissaro Bhikkhu's commentary on his translation of "Anapanasati Sutta: Mindfulness of Breathing" (*Access to Insight*, 25 September 2010, www.accesstoinsight.org/tipitaka/mn/mn.118.than.html).

whole of the visual field that appears before the eyes (not just an isolated object in it), the whole of the field of sounds (not just a single sound in the overall symphony), the whole of the mind (not just its most superficial dimension that is expressed through thought), and the whole of the body (not just one small part of it). And this is the terrain that we are ushered into by the practice of breathing through the whole body.

But what does "breathing through the whole body" actually mean? And how can we possibly breathe not just with the organs of respiration proper—the nose and mouth, the trachea, the bronchi, the lungs, the diaphragm, and the intercostal muscles—but also with the conscious participation of the entire body? And how and why does breathing in a way that involves the entire body have such a potent, transforming effect on consciousness itself?

These are the questions that this little book will attempt to answer.

PART ONE

THE FOUNDATION
OF THE BODY

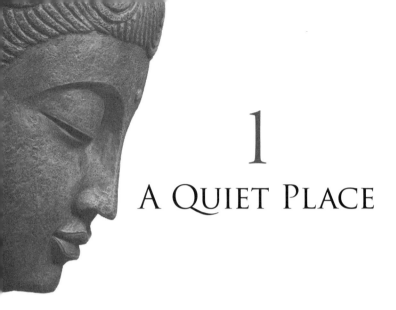

1

A Quiet Place

go to a quiet place in the wilderness,
the forest,
or even a room in an empty building

The opening instructions in each of the suttas tell us to go to a quiet place where we won't be disturbed: a wilderness location, a shady and protected spot in the forest perhaps, or even a quiet room in a building in which there's no other activity. If this was important in the time of the Buddha, you can imagine how much more important, and how much more difficult, it is for us today. There were no machines when the Buddha lived. No phones. No televisions. Music was a sublime rarity that could only be heard on special ceremonial occasions. Our modern soundscape is deafening in comparison.

When you hike into a mountain wilderness, you enter in

to a world of silence, an emptiness of sound punctuated only by the play of nature—wind rushing over rocks, water searching for a way down, the rhythmic thrum of bird's wings above your head. Silence is a sound that you feel with your body more than hear with your ear. You can feel its presence, but you don't really hear its absence. In many ways, the purpose of meditation practice is to help us find this place of silent presence within ourselves. When you sit down in a quiet place away from the commotion of the marketplace with its din of commerce and conversation, it becomes easier to drop down into the quiet place in the center of your body and mind.

The world and landscape of the Buddha don't exist anymore. Very few of us live an agrarian life in the country, and even so, contemporary country life is not immune to chain saws and tractors, lawn mowers and weed eaters, TV shows and iTunes, the whirring hum of a refrigerator, airplanes that pass miles above our heads. Even in the country, silence is a relative term at best. Living, as most of us do, in the middle of a city, presents even more challenges, but this doesn't mean that we can't meditate unless we travel to the mountains or live in the forest. In the context of modern life and the suttas both, it simply means that it is helpful to designate a place in our home as a sanctuary of silence, a corner where we won't be disturbed while we sit, a place where the phone can't reach us, a place where our children know not to bother us, preferably in a room whose door we can close behind us after we enter, a place for ourselves. It's quieter in there.

If things are not so noisy and distracting outside, it becomes easier to hear and feel what is going on inside. In a quiet place, we start hearing things we hadn't been hearing before and feeling things we hadn't been feeling before. One of the first things we may be surprised to notice when we sit down in meditation is how very noisy our mind is. Thoughts are constantly arising out of nowhere, one after the other, in a seemingly unbroken chain, like a radio host's monologue or a politician's filibuster, and they speak to us in a voice that, although muffled, sounds suspiciously like our own. In a quiet place, with our attention turned inward, away from any external tugs and pulls, we start hearing the unspoken chatter going on in our mind, which the noise of the world of commerce— and our participation in it—so effectively conceals.

Thoughts run on and on, and they are compelling (if monotonous and repetitive) storytellers, reminding us of things that have happened in the past, imagining things that might happen in the future. Thoughts let us reminisce about our past triumphs and failures and prepare us for whatever lies ahead, but they never let us experience the present moment. The present moment can only be felt into, never thought about. Our thoughts conceal the present moment from us.

When we begin to meditate, we often hope to discover that still, quiet place inside ourselves about which spiritual literature speaks so glowingly. But what we mostly discover instead, at least at first, is just how very unquiet we are. This realization is as important as it may be humbling or dismaying, because there's no way that we can quiet the mind unless we first become aware of how very noisy it is.

Sitting in a quiet place introduces us not only to the noise of a mind that can be too loud but also to the muted and muffled silence of a body that begs to be listened to. If the mind is like the guest who's too loud, self-absorbed, and occasionally out of control, the body is like a child who has taken the imperative to be seen but not heard to the extreme—overly silent, strangely absent, underactive, even vacant. Sitting in a quiet place, we start realizing that we don't feel the body very much at all, that we suppress the tactile world of sensation. The activity in every cell of the body generates sensations that we're capable of feeling, trillions upon trillions of sensations, little tactile blips that vibrate and oscillate at extraordinarily rapid rates of frequency. Massed together, these sensations form a shimmering field that can be felt to occupy the space of the entire body and even a bit beyond, pulsating, vibrating, tingling. But mostly we don't let ourselves feel much of the immense richness and variety of this great, loamy web of tactile life. We shut down its presence and turn off its feeling.

There's so much to feel that we hold ourselves back from feeling. There's so much to be aware of that thought conceals. When we sit down in our quiet place, no more racing here and there, no more tugs and pulls, we can turn our attention to the cycle of breath and start listening and feeling. Breathing in . . . breathing out . . . Maybe it will take minutes, or maybe it will take days or weeks, but mind does become quieter. Thoughts eventually do slow down. Sensations start coming out of hiding. Body begins to hum a bit.

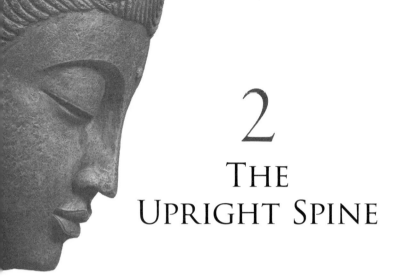

2
THE
UPRIGHT SPINE

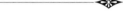

sitting down in a posture of meditation,
keeping the spine upright and erect

The purpose of meditation is to create the conditions that allow our illusory concepts of reality, and especially of how "I" fit into this picture, to drop away and be replaced instead by a direct experience of what's actually happening. However, even though the process of transformation that the Buddha urged us to undertake occurs at the very core of consciousness itself, we need to begin this quest by applying physics before psychology.

The Buddha's instructions on breathing begin by telling us to sit down with our spine erect and straight. In the time of the Buddha, to sit in meditation meant that you would sit down on the ground with your legs folded and crossed in front of you. Most meditators today still sit in a cross-legged posture but others have found it easier to sit in a kneeling position, either on a low, slanted bench or with a large pillow between their legs. For some people, especially in the West, who find sitting or kneeling on the floor too foreign, sitting on a chair is their preferred posture in which to meditate.

How you position your legs is much less important than what you do with your spine. Whether sitting cross-legged on the ground, kneeling on a bench or astride a cushion, or even sitting in a chair, the Buddha's instructions are very clear that you will want to sit up straight, your spine upright and balanced, not slumped forward, not leaning backward, not arching more to one side or the other.

To sit with an upright spine may seem like a simple enough request, but anyone who's ever attended an intensive meditation retreat knows how difficult this can be. If we force ourselves to sit up ramrod straight, like a soldier at attention, we bring tension into our posture, and breath becomes labored. If we sit without any awareness of the upright vertical, we tend to slump forward in our posture, and breath becomes imprisoned. The request to sit with an upright and erect spine is as challenging an instruction as any in the sutta.

Sitting with an upright and erect spine expresses a bearing of dignity and grace, but the purpose of the Buddha's instructions has nothing to do with aesthetics. It has more to do with the felt understanding of some of the most basic premises of Newtonian physics and the application of some of the most basic principles of structural engineering. Simply put, structures that are aligned along a predominantly vertical axis are supported by the force of gravity, while structures that are not so aligned have to create that support themselves.*

Architects, sculptors, and engineers from all ages (as well as any child who has ever built a snowman) have known that, if you want to build a tall, upright, and stable structure, then you need to make sure it is designed and constructed around a central vertical axis. While the discovery of materials of high tensile strength has allowed architects and engineers to vision and build ever taller skyscrapers, it is equally the flawless verticality of such structures that lets them attain their breathtaking heights. If each successive story of a skyscraper is balanced directly on top of the one beneath it, gravity secures the entire building, and there's no danger of it toppling over. Build a tall structure, however, with its shape veering away from the vertical, and you end up not with a functional building but with a tourist attraction like the Leaning Tower of Pisa, which has recently had to undergo major reinforcement to its foundation to keep it from eventually falling over and turning into a pile of rubble.

We can't escape gravity's pull. It is always and forever act-

---

*While modern physics has traveled far beyond Isaac Newton's original vision of gravity as a force that draws smaller objects to larger ones, replacing it instead with an understanding of how massive celestial bodies curve the space around them and catch smaller bodies in that curvature, Newton's original vision still works exceedingly well when applied to the scale of human beings living on the earth rather than to the unimaginably large sizes of the universe. Every time you throw an apple directly above you, it is going to come back down and hit you on the head, and it doesn't really matter a whole lot whether the bruise is the result of *the curvature of space* or *the force of gravity*. Newton's explanation for why the apple so unfailingly returns to earth is still extremely helpful for meditators seeking to figure out how to sit, how to breathe, and how to encounter the truth about themselves.

ing on us. However, what we can do is tend to the upright spine and organize the structure of the body around an upright vertical axis. Playing with upright balance in this way transforms gravity's pull from a force against which we have to constantly brace ourselves into a source of support and buoyancy that allows us to relax.

In contrast to the intrepid skyscrapers that dominate the skylines of our major cities, think for a moment of Fallingwater, the famous country home designed by the visionary twentieth-century architect Frank Lloyd Wright. Its cantilevered levels appear to float in space above the waterfall as they extend themselves audaciously outward from the central structure of the house. In order to achieve this form, engineers had to massively reinforce the cantilevered sections, binding them securely to the base structure of the house that rests on solid ground. If their proximate attachment weren't so securely reinforced, it would have been impossible for them to maintain their form, and they would have fallen over into the waterfall.

Now think of a person sitting in meditation. Many meditators sit in a posture reminiscent of Fallingwater, with their head and neck extending out precariously in front of the centerline of their torso. The musculature in their upper back and neck has to maintain constant tension to stabilize the neck and head, for if it were to truly relax, the head and neck would just drop forward and down onto the chest. If a sitting meditator doesn't pay attention to the Buddha's advice to sit up with a straight and erect spine, he or she will have to exert a significant degree of muscular tension to keep from toppling over, and such constant bracing and tension will obstruct the flow of breath through the body.

So the first thing the Buddha tells you to do when you sit down to meditate is to pay attention to the upright spine, the vertical line of the body, like a giant sequoia tree whose trunk is perfectly straight, whose roots sink deep into the earth, and whose topmost branches reach high into the sky. In order to sit in this way in a cross-legged posture, it is helpful to first place a thirty-inch-square cushioned mat on the floor or ground to soften the contact between the hard floor and your feet, ankles, and knees. On top, and to the rear, of this cushioning mat you will then want to place a smaller, supporting pillow or cushion on which to rest your buttocks. That allows you to create a stable triangular base of support, with your slightly raised buttocks and your two knees forming the angles of the triangle, over which the major segments of your upper torso—your belly, chest, shoulders, neck, and head—can line themselves up. A body that's upright and erect doesn't have to provide its support through the tensioning of its musculature. It can start to relax instead, and relaxation is the core principle on which the possibility of breathing through the whole body depends.*

Whether you experience gravity as friend or foe depends entirely on how much vertical alignment you bring to the structure of your sitting posture. Sitting in such a way that you need to fight with gravity locks you into a constant battle—which you can never win—and breeds tension in the body and contraction in the mind. Befriending gravity, receiving its gift of support, you can begin to let go and relax whatever you don't need to hold on to anymore.

_____

*For a more detailed analysis of the structural issues that support an erect and upright spine, the reader may want to look at the author's earlier book, *The Posture of Meditation* (Boston: Shambhala, 1996).

3
CENTER OF GRAVITY

One of my favorite toys as a child was an inflatable clown that appeared enormous to me, but probably stood only three or four feet tall. This clown had the shape of a highly exaggerated pear with a tiny, round head sitting on top of an overly large, bloated, round body. This rather strange shape made for a very stable toy and meant that an extremely boisterous young fellow like myself could unleash untold fury on this poor clown, pretending that he was my opponent in a heavyweight championship boxing match, whacking him repeatedly on the head so that he would fall over every time, only to immediately bounce back fully upright with the smile on his face undiminished!

The secret of this clown's remarkable ability to take a punch and spring right back up from the canvas was that it had a very low center of gravity. As aspiring meditators, there's much for us to learn from the example of this clown (including the undeterred smile on its face). What this toy primarily has to teach us, though, is the value of lowering our center of gravity from our head down into our heart and belly.

Sitting with an upright and erect spine, we start relaxing tensions in our body and mind through the simple gesture of surrendering the weight of the body to the pull of gravity. As our weight drops downward, our felt center of gravity drops downward with it, but still we remain upright. Were a meditator who sits in a slumped posture to let go and relax the tensions in her body in the same way, she would fall forward onto her mat and, unlike the resilient clown, not bounce right back up again and certainly not with a smile on her face.

The center of gravity in most humans today is situated high up in the head, just the opposite of the clown of my childhood. It is here where we predominantly experience our self to exist; not coincidentally, it is here where the mind spins its web of thoughts. So thorough is our conventional identification with the speaker of our thoughts who lives in our head that some of us have little, if any, awareness of the body from the neck down.

Lost in thought, we get drawn up into our head, and our body becomes top heavy. Surrendering our weight to the pull of gravity, however, while releasing tension, we drop back down into the body, right into the center of its felt presence, and the body again becomes more stable. This lowering of the center of gravity is emphasized in some Chinese and Japanese schools of Buddhism through their insistence on dropping one's mind into the *tan tien* or the *hara,* which are located in the lower belly. These schools teach that the journey of awakening starts in the thoughts in the head and ends in the presence in the belly. To sink and settle deeper into oneself is to be drawn down into this more stable center of gravity.

The effects of the inability to relax go beyond the physical creation of pain or numbness, generalized discomfort, and an inefficiency of movement that hampers the grace and ease of the body. Patterns of unnecessary myofascial holding and tension also limit the mind and our sense of self to their most superficial dimensions of expression through fueling the constant parade of involuntary thoughts. Dissolving thought back into presence is no different from relaxing tension anywhere in the body. We can surrender the weight of thought to gravity's omnipresent pull. We can drop it by letting go of the tension that fosters and sustains it. As the tensions behind the thought relax, we drop back down into our own center of gravity where thoughts don't intrude as often.

The importance of relaxing the body and mind in the process of meditation can't be overemphasized, and this relaxation inevitably results in the lowering of your center of gravity. Sitting in meditation, you become like the clown of my youth—stable, secure, always smiling, always picking yourself up from the ground after falling down over and over again. As the Japanese Buddhist teacher Sasaki Roshi is fond of saying: "Buddha *is* the center of gravity." To find the center of gravity in yourself is to relax completely and lower it down into the heart and belly where it is more naturally at home. And once you start relaxing and settling down into yourself in this way, it becomes much easier to breathe.

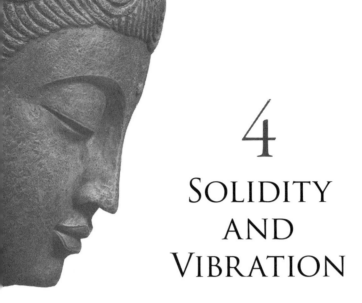

4

SOLIDITY
AND
VIBRATION

Ordinarily we think of the body as solid matter and the self that inhabits the body as a very concrete entity. The body, however, is not solid at all. In the first place, it is composed primarily of water, so much so that a prominent anatomist once wryly speculated that human beings were but a clever strategy on the part of water to move itself from place to place. As much as 70 percent of the body is made up of fluid liquids while only the remaining 30 percent is composed of minerals of the earth.

If we were to refine this analysis even further and examine individual atoms of a human cell under a high-powered microscope, we would suddenly be faced with a world that more closely resembles a miniature version of our solar system, with tiny dots of matter separated by vast amounts of empty space. Taken as a whole, the mass of the body is mostly empty space with the occasional smattering of tiny particles floating through it. And then, if we were to focus even further on these tiny particles, we would see that they appear not at all as solid matter but as vibratory phenomena, constantly moving, flickering on and off as they appear and disappear throughout the etheric space of the body.

Mostly, however, we don't directly experience the body as it is. We don't tune in to its shimmery, vibratory nature. We don't feel the minute, flickering sensations that exist in every cell. Instead, we stay lodged in our mind from whose perspective we assume that our body, like all the other convincingly solid objects we view in our environment, must be solid as well. But if we give ourselves permission to truly start experiencing our body, to really feel it, every little part of it, everything dissolves into shimmer and vibration.

We can never experience the body as solid. We can only conceive of it that way, and conceptualization is a function of a mind that works best when undisturbed by the awareness of the body. Engaged in thought, like a balloon floating upward, we raise our center of gravity high into our head, and the feeling ground of the body becomes smaller, further away, a distant vision. Body keeps the mind tethered to the present moment, but it has to be directly experienced as sensation and not just thought about as object.

When we sit with an upright and erect spine, relaxing the tensions of the body by surrendering its weight to the pull of gravity, lowering our center of gravity back into our heart and belly, we're better able to experience body as it is, and what we find is a field phenomenon of minute vibrations—constantly shimmering, changing, flickering—suspended in a matrix of space. And anything that we still experience as somewhat solid and dense gradually reveals itself as muscular tension and holding, as resistance to gravity, to the current of the life force, and to the process of relaxation. Once real relaxation is felt, it is impossible not to remain drawn to its feeling. If we come across an area in the body that feels tense and solid, we naturally start allowing it to relax and let go; once that happens, we're left living in a body that is even more insubstantial: just vibration, just space.

So much for our idea of being a solid body. But what about the belief that *who I am* is some kind of stable entity, that at the very center and core of my body I exist as an unchanging reference point, at least throughout the life of this body, and that what I call *me* is actually what I am? To be honest, nothing seems more natural than to view ourselves in this way. However, if we examine our sense of self in the same way we just looked at the body, we may be surprised to discover that the self we conventionally view as decidedly intact and stable is about as substantial as our body is solid, which is to say, not very much at all. The solidity of the body and the substantiality of the self are convenient conceptions that allow us to live in the world, but they don't accurately describe the truth of our essential nature.

Where do you exist?

"Up in my head," you say.

And how do you know that?

"Well, I can feel *myself* there, and I'm the entity that's thinking all these thoughts; I'm the speaker of the monologue that's going on and on inside my head."

Fair enough (and once again, let's be honest: this sounds right as rain). But if you really start turning your attention to your sense of self, beginning by zeroing in on where you feel it in your body, then probing that place, feeling into it deeper and deeper, examining what's actually happening from moment to moment, the concrete nature of the individual self may start becoming significantly less substantial than you ordinarily believe it to be.

So accustomed have we become to this notion that *who I am* is an entity named *I* who inhabits the physical body in which *I* live that we rarely, if ever, take an honest look to determine whether it is actually all that accurate. And when we do, especially in a relaxed and upright body, that notion starts coming apart like a house of cards. Just as our "solid" body is felt as vibratory shimmer, our "stable" mind and sense of self get deconstructed down into a rapidly flashing procession of thoughtforms and self-images, constantly changing and shifting, appearing, disappearing, nothing stable, nothing lasting for longer than a moment, just a process of change.

Our conventional sense of self is closely aligned with, and powerfully reinforced by, the process of linguistic thinking. Our language names us as the speaker of our thoughts, and one of its primary purposes is to draw distinctions between things. That's what a name is: a signal to point out a specific object, feeling, or event in contrast to everything that it isn't. Sufi teachers and poets often speak of the troubles and suffering of *separation,* a word that references this felt notion that *who I am* lives as a kind of floating island in the sea of the universe, a tiny and minuscule speck separate and distinct from everything that I can perceive to exist outside of the physical body that I identify with (but don't experience). In contrast to this felt sense of separation is our natural state or what the Sufis call *union,* a condition as equally palpable and real as the felt sense of separation but totally opposite from it in terms of its effect on consciousness.

Separation spawns feelings of uneasiness, loneliness, alienation, fear; union welcomes us back into an embrace of inclusiveness, joining, merging. The underlying feeling tone of separation is one of painful compression, as though too much sensation is being asked to occupy too small a space; the feeling tone of union is one of relief and flow, as though a logjam in our body and mind has been suddenly cleared.

The Sufis tell us that to undertake this journey from separation to union one very important thing is necessary: we have to dissolve and give up the unrelentingly apparent solidity of the self and our absolute identification with it. The word *I* is a mark of differentiation, a signifier of distinction, a signpost that separates the world into everything *me* and everything *not me*. But this demarcation and separation, say the Sufis, is exactly what causes all our troubles, our fears, our bodily pains; it is what happens when a concept that we hold to be true distorts the reality it purports to reflect.

Probing your thinking mind and sense of self, examining what's actually happening moment to moment, you begin to see how they're supported by patterns of tension and holding in the physical body. When you become lost in thought, you unwittingly contract the energies in your cranium, and you do this by bringing tension into the intricate web of the musculature that shapes and supports your head. Relaxing the tensions in your head, deep inside your cranium, in your eyes, your jaws, your temples, your throat and mouth, you take away the ground in which thought takes root. As thoughts dissolve, your formerly very solid sense of self as this entity named *I* (we all have exactly this same pet name for ourselves) starts coming undone as well.

The body is just space and vibration, but you can only experience this when you're deeply relaxed. And when you do experience this bodily state, what happens to *you*? Where do *you* go? And what is it that replaces the *you* of tension when real relaxation supplants the holding and resistance of imbalance?

5

STILLNESS
AND MOTION

Ours is a universe in which everything moves. Electrons spin in their orbits around the nucleus of atoms like whirling dervishes turning around a sacred center, unable to stop. Subatomic particles that create the stuff of matter play a never-ending game of hide and seek—now appearing, now disappearing, now reappearing again, but sometimes in an entirely different location in space. The universe itself is constantly on the move, expanding ever outward to a destination that no one can predict. Stillness is but a relative term at best, an abstract concept and idea; in real life it doesn't exist.

As important as it is to establish an upright spine, it is even more important to understand that the upright spine is a moving spine and that subtle movements can occur between each and every vertebra, even at every joint of the body, on every inhalation and exhalation of the breath. To understand how to breathe through the whole body as the Buddha suggested, nothing is more helpful than to recognize that, in a deeply relaxed body, the force of breath can cause the entire body to remain in a state of subtle, constant motion.

The first thing I invariably notice when I look out over a roomful of sitting meditators is how overly still almost everyone is holding themselves. Granted, the practice *is* relatively still, certainly in comparison to more physically active exercises like dance and sport. But as a value applied to the practice of meditation, stillness refers only to a quality of mind, not to a rigid and frozen body. Sitting in meditation, relaxing . . . subtle movements can be felt throughout the entire body in response to each and every breath. When we allow these natural motions to occur, mind becomes calmer and sensations come more alive. But if we brace ourselves against them, mind gets stirred and body loses touch with itself.

Certainly one of the genuine benefits that comes with the practice of sitting meditation—regardless of the tradition you belong to or the technique you're exploring—is simply in learning how to sit and relax and forego the impulse and urgency to jump up and move about, in both body and thought. However, this quest to still the fidgeting impulses of the body and mind quickly reaches a point of diminishing returns if you start believing that an inner stillness of mind is somehow dependent on an outer stillness of body and so begin to freeze and hold the body as though you were trying to emulate a stone garden statue of the Buddha.

The body is constantly on the move. It moves through space as it walks across a room. It shimmers and vibrates at the level of the cells. Deeply relaxed, it can be felt to pulsate and throb to the organic rhythms of the heartbeat, the breath, the nerve signals racing through their fibers, the flowing rivers of blood and lymph. Nothing still.

At least so long as the body can keep relaxing its tensions, that is. Tension in the body always causes some degree of stillness at its nearest joint, and areas of frozen stillness always resist the force of the breath that wants to pass through that part of the body.

Simply put, when you tense your body, you become still; when you relax your body, everything can start to move again in resilient response to the natural flow of the breath. The upright spine, through the play of balance, allows you to begin to relax; surrendering to the inherent motion in all things by allowing resilient movement to occur throughout the body in response to the breath allows relaxation to continue.

The action of breath is initiated through the repetitive contraction and relaxation of the diaphragm, the dome-shaped muscle that separates our chest cavity from our abdomen. It functions as a pump that draws oxygen-rich air into our body on the inhalation and expels the waste products of respiration on every exhalation. Every time the diaphragm contracts, air gets suctioned into our body through our nose or mouth. Every time the diaphragm relaxes, used air gets pushed out, and this pumping motion is repeated over and over and over again throughout our entire life.

The rhythmic contraction and relaxation of the diaphragm generate a propulsive force not unlike the force that causes waves to move through a body of water. Just as the force that creates waves in the ocean causes movement to occur through the entire body of water through which it is passing, so can the force of breath generate movement throughout the entire physical body so long as the body remains fluid and relaxed. It is impossible to imagine the force that creates waves in the ocean *not* causing motion to occur in the water, but what we tend to do is resist the force of the breath by introducing tension into the musculature, effectively freezing the body at its joints.

Imagine for a moment a pool table on which all fifteen balls are arranged in a perfectly straight line with a quarter inch of space between them. If you were to place the cue ball a few feet away on the same line, and strike it so it squarely hit the first ball in the row, what would happen? The force generated by the contact between the cue ball and the first ball would be transferred along and through the entire row of balls to ultimately cause the ball at the end of the line to bounce away.

Now think of the bones of the body as being like the line of billiard balls, in close contact with each other at the joints, and think of the contraction of the diaphragm initiating the cycle of breath as the striking of the cue ball. On a pool table, the force of that strike gets transferred through the entire line of balls. In a completely relaxed body, the contracting force and motions of breath can be transferred from one joint of the body to the next until it is transmitted through the entire body. On the exhalation, every little part of the body relaxes back to where it began. In this way the whole body stays in constant motion, expanding and contracting, from one breath to the next and to the next.

But what happens if a joint in the body refuses to participate in the wavelike motion, refuses to respond to the transmitted force of the breath that strikes it? The only way it could resist the force of the breath would be through tensing the tissues around the joint. In the image of the pool table, it would be as though one of the pool balls had been glued to the felt surface. The transmitted motion of the breath would get stopped in its tracks at that resistant joint and travel no farther.

While stillness—and resistance to the force of the breath—can exist anywhere in the body, it is particularly evident in the head and neck. When we hold our head still in meditation, we draw tension into the upper back, the neck, and the cranium, and this pattern of tension keeps feeding our thoughts. To the extent, then, that we so stiffen the musculature of the neck that our head becomes completely unmoving and unwavering, we inadvertently support the very process of semiconscious thought that our meditation practice wants to help us slow down, perhaps even dissolve, certainly at least dis-identify with, so that we can start accessing levels of mind that exist underneath the thoughts.

Sitting in meditation in an upright and relaxed body, breath blows, and the body, every little part of it, can respond. Each vertebra can shift its angle and distance from its immediate neighbors on every inhalation . . . and on every exhalation . . . So can each bone. As the force of breath keeps passing through the length of the body, the head can start bobbing up and down and back and forth, ever so subtly, just like a fishing bobber floating on top of the surface of a lake over which a breeze is blowing. When the body moves naturally like this, the mind starts slowing down. Exposed to the constant, gentle motions of the body, the inner monologue doesn't have as stable a stage on which to stand and broadcast its views.

When the fatherly god of the Old Testament disapproved of the behavior of the Israelites, he would often express his displeasure by uttering a most unusual imprecation: he would call them a "stiff-necked people." What might a stiff neck signify in an Old Testament context? Resistance, stubbornness perhaps. The refusal or unwillingness to see the truth clearly. Love of self over respect toward elders and community. Disobedience. Just the kinds of things that authoritarian dads don't like to see in their children.

When we sit down to meditate, we do so to give up our resistances, to align ourselves obediently with the laws of nature, to soften our unrelenting sense of individual self. We sit so we can start seeing things as they are, rather than through the distorting lens of our beliefs and prejudices. And yet, to the extent that we get lost in thought (which we do on a maddeningly regular basis), we too are stiff-necked people. If you start paying close attention to the correlation between thought and body, you'll begin to notice how the process of thought—especially the involuntary thoughts and rambling inner monologues—is always accompanied by a head that's held still, and the primary way you hold the head still is to stiffen the musculature of the neck.

Breath wants to liberate itself, to free itself from the encasing and confining prison of the body's frozen stillness. It is as though the body has been built up and created from multiple layers of different tissues and organs, all superimposed one on top of the other like strips of papier-mâché. Unlike the dried and hardened strips of papier-mâché, however, the layers of the body are composed of living tissue, and living tissue—like the waters of the ocean—wants to move in response to the forces and sources of motion that animate it. The whole of the body wants to keep moving, constantly, resiliently moving, in surrendered response to the force of the breath that wants to breathe through it. Layers of tissue want to move and flow freely and smoothly over one another as the force of the breath passes through them, everything moving freely, floating on the breath, not even a single little part of the body left behind, everything in motion, just like the universe.

6

LETTING GO

The primary action of meditation is not really an action at all. It is less something that we do than something that we undo. It is more of a relaxing, an allowing, a yielding to, a letting go of the held patterns of tension and contraction that keep us confined in bodies that cry out for release and minds that get stuck in thought.

We can't heroically force these patterns of tension and contraction to change. We can't do battle with them in hopes of vanquishing or subduing or just plain wiping them out. We can't force the body back to life or the mind to become still. It doesn't work that way. The most profitable thing we can do is to give ourselves permission to feel what's here to be felt exactly as it is and then relax into that feeling through a gesture of letting go.

Letting go is like a sudden eruption of relaxation that spreads through the body, releasing tension everywhere it touches. Tensions in the body and mind only become stagnant and fixed when we protect ourselves from feeling them or forcibly attempt to change them. Both these attitudes effectively block our ability to feel, and not until tension is felt deeply does it stand a chance of letting go, dropping away, transforming itself back into shimmer or presence.

The letting go that initiates a breath that breathes through the whole body occurs through a sudden dropping of the weight of the body, which feels a bit like freefalling through space. Just let go to gravity's tug as though a stone were dropping through the middle of your spine way down deep into the interior of the earth, and coordinate this sensation of dropping with the onset of inhalation. As you do this, resilient movement can start entering again into held areas of tension and contraction. This gentle movement through the body acts like the lapping of water over sandstone rocks. The more movement in the current of the river that flows over the sandstone, the quicker the stone will dissolve away; the more the whole body participates in the motions of breath, the quicker tension is released.

Through this simple, natural gesture of letting go, breath rushes in and sets the body in motion, expanding into the belly and through the torso on the inhalation, settling back and retracing its steps on the exhalation. Like a sailboat riding on the wind, up and down the troughs of the waves, the body stays in constant motion, not by forcing itself to move, but simply by letting go. As the weight of the body and the heft of the mind are surrendered to gravity, the force of the breath moves through the entire length of the body however it likes.

So whenever you become aware in your practice that you've gone off course or gotten stuck on a shoal, that you've gotten lost in a thought, that you've started holding on, bracing yourself, bringing contraction into your body and mind, just remember to let go again in the most casual, non-forced way possible. Tensions relax, the chatter of the mind slows down, and breath has no choice but to breathe through more of the body.

This constant returning of awareness to feeling and the possibility of letting go is the corrective course of meditation. Everything else is allowing and surrender. A hundred times during an hour's sitting the mind sneaks in like a cat burglar, steals your awareness away without you even knowing, takes you off on a thought journey during which you forget all about breath, about body, even about vision and sound. During these journeys, breath gets more tied up and body becomes more frozen. And then, a hundred times an hour, you wake up to the intrusion and bring your awareness back to the possibilities of letting go again.

Sometimes the letting go feels like sand falling through your fingers. Other times it's more tentative. And at other times still it may cause you to tremble. You just keep letting go, as best you can, breath by breath by breath. What could be more simple? What could be more challenging?

Every breath you take offers you a clear choice: either you let go, surrender to, and cooperate with the force of the breath, or you brace yourself to resist it. We've all learned how to restrict the breath, how to keep it, and ourselves, held back and contained. Bringing the attitudes of relaxation and letting go into our meditation practice, we invite the motions of breath back into more and more of the body.

PART TWO

THE BREATH
OF UNENDING
MOTION

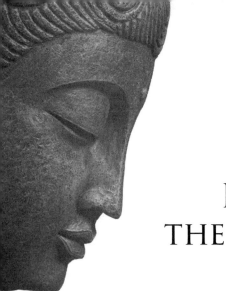

7

INTO
THE CENTER

begin by observing the breath in the front of the body

remain aware as you breathe in
remain aware as you breathe out

notice if the breath is long or short

as you breathe in, breathe in through the whole body
as you breathe out, breathe out through the whole body

The Buddha's instructions on breathing describe a natural progression that begins with the simplest observation of the action of breath, becomes ever more refined in its discernment of the nuances of breathing, and ultimately ends in a sophisticated merging with the breath that effectively integrates mind, body, and breath into a unified phenomenon.

Because breathing is such an involuntary function, we mostly pay it little attention. After all, breath comes and goes on its own, so why give it any energy or pay it any notice? Buddhism's simple response to this is that paying attention to respiration—locating it, observing it, probing it, surrendering to it, and finally merging with it—helps us awaken from the ideas, concepts, and dreamy notions we hold about ourselves into a more directly felt truth of who we are (the term *buddha* means "one who has woken up"). Breath always and only happens right now. We can record our past history and look forward to a future yet to come, but this moment is the only moment in which life actually takes place. Remaining aware of the passage of breath helps us stay more grounded and embodied, right now, always in this moment.

Understanding both how potently effective the practice of breath awareness is and just how unaware we ordinarily are of this most basic of bodily functions, the Buddha created a roadmap of the breath that tells us where to begin, how to proceed, and what our destination might look like. It's a journey that starts out at the periphery of awareness and moves progressively deeper into the center of our body, our being, our mind. By following his sequence of directions, we keep traveling back down into our self, ever further inside, always deeper, right into the very center of our center.

Because we ordinarily have little awareness of the passage of breath, the Buddha begins by instructing us to start locating it at the front of the body where it can be the most easily noticed and felt. The air we breathe first comes into contact with the front of the body as it passes over our nostrils on its journey into our lungs. Like a watchman standing guard at the walled gate of a city, carefully checking out everyone who enters or leaves, we can fix our entire attention on the entrance to our nostrils and simply pay, as best we can, close and concentrated attention to every breath we take as it enters and leaves the main breathing gate of the body.

To observe the action of breath in this way, all you're asked to do is stay aware of the sensations that breath creates as it touches the nostrils on its passage in and out of the body. Like a breeze blowing back and forth across the surface of a pond, the inhalation can be felt as a cool, rushing flow of sensations, while the exhalation, emerging from the heated environment of the body, is much warmer. Cooling air rushes into the body while warming air leaves, and the only place you can experience this contrast in temperature and alternation of directional flow is at the very front of the body at the entrance to the nostrils.*

In addition to the nostrils, there's another place at the front of the body that other Buddhist schools instruct their students to focus on. No matter how still a meditator may be sitting, there will always be some discernible movement in the belly in response to the contraction and relaxation of the diaphragm. When the diaphragm contracts on the inhalation, the belly can

---

*From the time of the early Greek philosophers right up through the Renaissance, the prevailing Western theory of why we breathe was almost entirely based on this felt difference in temperature between the inhalation and exhalation. Breath was thought to function as a kind of radiator that kept the furnace of the heart from overheating: the inhalation cooled the heat of the heart, like water poured on a fire; the exhalation released the heated air, like steam rising.

be felt to rise and expand. When it relaxes on the exhalation, the belly can be felt to fall and settle back down.

Practices that instruct you to remain aware of the passage of breath by fixing your attention either at the nostrils or the belly accord with the Buddha's opening instructions to observe the breath at the front of the body. In Southeast Asia, the widely popular breathing practices of *anapanasati* focus almost entirely on these first instructions. The meditator starts by fixing all of his (or her) attention on the activity of the breath in either of these two locations at the front of the body. Then, once he realizes that he's lost awareness of the breath, that the mind has wandered off into thought, he gently returns his attention back to the nostrils or belly. The practice is potent: over long hours, days, and weeks, strong concentration is developed, and the mind becomes calmer and clearer.

However, the instructions in the sutta don't end with the opening suggestion to keep your attention focused at the front of the body. Once you've spent some time locating the breath at the nostrils or the belly, you can start narrowing your lens, focusing on breath's subtler textures, while also widening your lens to include more of it. To do this, the next instructions in the sutta imply that you take a step backward into the mystery space of the body that exists behind the nostrils and the surface wall of the belly. It is as though the vigilant watchman at the gate, instead of just remaining glued to his post and duty, observing whoever enters and leaves, starts accompanying each visitor as a personal chaperone, walking at their side as they move into the town center, conduct their business, leave their mark on the city, are changed forever, and then leave.

To more fully understand the phenomenon of breath, you'll want to become aware not just of what it feels like as it enters and leaves the body through the nose or the mouth but how it can be felt to pass down the trachea, enter and fill the lungs, how it then turns around and reverses its path. You'll want to feel how the pulsing motions of breath aren't just limited to the outer wall of the belly but can be felt to radiate through the abdomen and torso. Broadening your focus in this way, you start experiencing so much more of the intimate dance of breath and body and of the sensations that the partners in this dance routinely kick up. No two breaths, like no two snowflakes, are ever exactly alike. They may be longer or shorter than one another, fuller or slighter. They may be labored, or they may be free. They may feel like silk passing over silk or they may be rough and coarse, and there are thousands of varieties of silk and thousands of subtly different ways to be rough or coarse.

The Buddha's shorthand instructions are simply to notice if the breath is long or short, but the implication is that it is time now to move literally deeper into the examination of the breath. In order to deepen your understanding and feeling awareness of the breath, you have to go inside your body where the true activity of breathing takes place, right down into the primary organs of respiration. The breath starts at the nostrils but then drops down into the windpipe, branches out into the bronchi, and starts filling the lungs. What happens along that pathway as breath passes through? What happens at the height of the inhalation? Is there a momentary pause that separates the phases of inhalation and exhalation, or is there just an imperceptible shift that turns the inhalation right around into the exhalation, and vice versa? What do you feel, and where do you feel it, as the impulse to breathe causes the diaphragm to contract and the belly to rise? What happens in your belly, your back, your upper torso when the diaphragm relaxes? How strong or shallow is the breath that enters and leaves the body? Is the breath long, or is it short? There's no shortage of details that can be paid attention to and felt.

Every breath we take, round after round, stimulates distinct sensations along the entire pathway of respiration. The rising and falling of the belly and the sensations at the nostrils are just the distal ends of the spectrum of breath, and there's a lot going on in the space between them. Every inhalation can be felt to pass deep into the interior of the body, in a wave of sensations, as it moves along and into the passages and chambers of the respiratory system. As breath turns around to pass back out of the body, the wave recedes.

Paying attention to the breath in this way makes the scholars who argue whether the instructions in the sutta refer to breathing through the entire physical body or only through the entire body of the breath both right. Here, in this intermediate step, we start feeling more of the whole body of the breath. We feel it as it moves into the body; we feel what happens as it leaves. All along the pathway of respiration, we can hitch ourselves to the breath, riding on it like a miner to descend into the depths of the lungs and float back out with it as it is expelled on the exhalation. In this way, we start blurring the boundaries that ordinarily separate our inner and outer worlds. With every breath we take, we invite the outer world deep inside the body, feel how it transforms us, then how it leaves the interior of the body and passes out again.

While the opening instructions to remain aware of the breath at either the nostrils or the belly can help develop strong concentration in the meditator, the subsequent instructions about breath are not so much exercises in concentration as invitations to go deeper. As you keep on observing the subtleties of breath over long hours, days, and weeks, you're naturally led to follow it down into the body's interior.

But the awareness of breath's passage into the body needn't stop at the bottom of the lungs any more than at the entrance to the nostrils or the surface of the belly. As breath and awareness both become more refined, and as body continues to relax, you start feeling how breath doesn't just interact with the organs of respiration proper but how its motions can be felt to spread through, affect, and touch the entire body, every little part of it, every joint of it, every cell of it. It's not just a function of the nostrils or the belly. It's not just a function of the respiratory system. You can feel it everywhere now, the entire body an organ of breathing, the entire body breathing in, the entire body breathing out, like the expansion and contraction of an amoeba, inherent motion through the entire organism. You can feel it in your arms, in your legs, in your head, torso, and pelvis, in every cell of your body; you can feel it in the subtle, yielding motions at relaxed joints.

In reality, breath and body are so intimately related that it is difficult to isolate or even speak of one in the absence of the other. One is always a direct reflection of the other, and at their core they can never be separated. If your awareness of body is limited, breath will likewise be limited and restrained. If you're able to relax into the feeling presence of the body, breath comes alive, and it can be felt to stimulate sensation and responsive motion through more and more of the body. If you undertake a truly thorough examination of the breath, you will have to keep expanding your field of observation until you arrive at a place where breath and body start merging into a unified phenomenon, just as is indicated in the sutta's concluding instructions to breathe through the whole body.

The three levels of breath that the Buddha speaks of—starting at the front of the body, moving into the interior of the body, and finally spreading through the whole of the body—correspond to three deepening layers of what we experience our self to be. Moving from one to the next to the next is like going on an archaeological dig of our body and mind. Starting out at the surface of the body where we feel very little, we dig down deeper into the interior, and finally reach the very center of our body from where we can feel everything all at once.

The quality of consciousness that passes as normal in the world at large is primarily a disembodied consciousness in which we often spend a good deal of time lost in thought. Divorced from the feeling ground of the body, mind tends to create self-images or personas that reflect who we think ourselves to be. The self-image is like a mask (the word *persona* comes from the Latin word for "mask") that we wear when we interact with the world. The masks may change depending on the situation (friendly, confrontational, neutral), but to varying degrees they're always there whenever we muffle the felt reality of the body. This quality of mind then generally identifies itself with the mask it has created, believing this mask to be *who I am,* wanting the world to believe this as well, and effectively forgetting that there may be other dimensions of experience that lie underneath it.

Where does a mask sit? Right on the front of our body, of course, and to the extent that we identify with our mask, the center of what we experience as our self can be felt in front of the body, not in it. Identified with our self-image, we lose awareness of the felt reality of our interior and have little choice but to believe ourselves to be the speaker of the stream of unbroken thoughts that passes through our mind. Identified with our self-image, we live our life as though it were a masked ball at which we go about our frivolities, never exposing the truth of who we are, interacting with others through the picture we've painted on our face. Buddhist teachers who speak about the importance of finding our *original face* want to help us take off our mask and find out what it has been covering up.

While it is often useful, and even wise, to interact with the outside world through the self-image we project at our surface, what the symbol of a mask underscores is that many of us, much of the time, aren't settled into the felt reality of the body. We hover instead at the periphery of the body where sensations can't touch us. The image of the mask suggests that we reside just in front of the body, and so it only makes sense that this is where the Buddha tells us to begin our observation of the cycle of the breath.

But then the instructions go deeper. We are told to start paying attention to the fuller range of sensations, qualities, and motions associated with the breath, and the only way we can do this is to go deeper into the awareness of our body's interior. Following breath all the way into the body, we inevitably go deeper into our self as well. Lost in thought, we lose awareness of our self, of the part of us that knows and feels that we exist.

Moving back inside, we reconnect with our self. This more conscious feeling of self-knowing (which is often first felt as a presence right behind the eyes in the interior of the cranium) is a more awakened place from which to function. Feeling and knowing our self in this moment, thoughts start fading, and when thoughts recede in this way, it becomes harder to get tangled up and lost in them.

Probing the reality that can be felt to exist underneath the topmost layer in which you identify with an image you've created of yourself, you move deeper and start contacting the actual felt experience of being a human, alive at this moment in time on the planet. Yes, that's me! And I'm awake to myself. And then the instructions go deeper still. Keep on refining your awareness of how breath and body interact during every phase of the breath, for as you do, you come to realize how no part of the body need be left out or uninvolved in the action of breathing, how breath can be felt to reach into and touch every little part of the body.

Starting off from a place in front of the body where you may often find yourself lost in thought, moving deeper into the interior of your body as you become more familiar with the subtleties of breath and of your self as well, arriving at a place where breath, body, and mind so line up that they start merging into a single, unified phenomenon—this is the pilgrimage that breath takes you on, down through successive layers of your self, from unconsciousness to consciousness to sciousness (William James's word for "essential nature").*

---

*My understanding of William James and his doctrine of sciousness, which some people liken to the nondual doctrines of Advaita Vedanta, comes from *Sciousness,* by Jonathan Bricklin.

First you need to know the self. Only then can it evolve beyond itself. As the solidity and stillness of the body give way to vibratory presence and resilient motion, the hard edges and implosive energies of the self of separation start softening and releasing as well. As the apparent solidity of the body melts, mind can melt along with it.

In the sutta, the Buddha isn't so much teaching breath techniques to be explored in sequence as describing a natural, organic progression that occurs for anyone who sets out on the journey of observing and understanding the relationship between breath, body, and mind. Starting out from a place with little awareness of the breath, you keep moving toward a place where you become indistinguishable from it.

8

THE KOAN
OF BREATHING

---

as you breathe in, breathe in through the whole body
as you breathe out, breathe out through the whole body

The Buddha often spoke in simple, pithy statements that are less like step-by-step instructions than they are like *koans,* or riddles, which we need to figure out for ourselves from the scantest of clues. In the Rinzai school of Zen Buddhism, meditators spend long hours focusing their mind on essentially alogical statements or stories called koans that make no sense whatsoever but are nonetheless presented as a kind of riddle or puzzle to which the meditator has to come up with an answer or, at least, a response.* The above-quoted sentences from the

---

*For example: *Shuzan held out his short staff and said, "If you call this a short staff, you oppose its reality. If you do not call it a short staff, you ignore the fact. Now what do you wish to call this?"*

Satipatthana Sutta are very much like a koan, except that we need to figure out this puzzle not with our mind but through the feeling awareness of our body.

Just as no one can provide you with the answer to a Zen koan, no one can show you definitively how to breathe through your whole body. You have to figure out on your own, by yourself, what you have to do (and mostly undo), and how you can best go about doing that. Breathing through your whole body is not in any way an expertise to attain or a skill set to perfect. It's not some far-off goal to achieve, but the possibility in the very breath you're taking, a constant reminder simply to let go as best you can, to relax into your body, to yield to the primal impulse to breathe. From one stepping-stone of breath to the next, it leads you along a path whose only goal is to be as present as possible to the possibilities of the stepping-stone you're on.

Focusing awareness on the breath at the front of the body is an instruction that's relatively easy to understand and follow. So are the implications of the suggestion to observe whether the breath is long or short. But breathing through the whole body is an entirely different kind of instruction. It's more like the answer to the riddle of breath than the instructions on how to solve it.

Breathing through the whole body hints at a condition in which body, breath, and mind—ordinarily so disconnected from one another—can be felt to come together into a single, coterminous phenomenon. While you have to discover for yourself how the integration of these three aspects of experience might occur, the following principles, and the exercises that follow, can help guide you in your efforts.

For starters, the practice is not about making any efforts, but about letting go. You can't artificially manufacture a breath that breathes through the whole body; nor would you want to. You can only surrender to the impulse to breathe and keep letting go, as best you can, of whatever tension and stillness you encounter in your body as you do. Letting go of whatever binds your body and contracts your mind is meditation's constant opportunity (as well as its challenge). Exploring the possibility of breathing through your whole body, you have no choice but to keep letting go.

The Buddha tells us that, before we begin focusing on the activity of the breath, we want to make sure that the spine is erect and upright. Don't, however, do yourself the disservice of believing there's a goal of some kind of perfected condition of balance and upright alignment that you need to attain and then maintain. Your goal isn't to mold your body into some idealized shape like pressing dough into a cookie cutter; your goal is simply to play with balance in the body you bring to the cushion, to feel how the sensations and energies in the body keep lightening up as the segments of the body keep lining up, one above the other. Playing with balance in meditation is always about remembering to let go into the next least effortful place.

Tensions in the body always function as a concealing blanket that covers over the felt life of the body's sensations, so as you begin to relax and let go, dropping the weight of the body through the upright spine, the feeling presence of the body emerges more and more. The more of your body you feel, the more opportunities you have to let go through the breath. Breath can only breathe through a body in touch with itself.

Just as sensation is everywhere, so is movement everywhere. Motions of breath and presence of body are inextricably linked. You can't have one without the other. A breath that breathes through the whole body will be a breath of constant, tidal motion.

Playing with balance, relaxing the body by surrendering its weight to gravity, opening to the possibility of feeling sensation in every cell of the body, letting go of tension in the body and contraction in the mind, opening to the subtle motions that want to occur in the body even as you sit silently on your cushion: these are the rules of thumb, the guiding principles that you want to keep circling back to over and over and over again as you explore the koan to breathe through the whole body. Each principle on its own implies or leads directly to the others. Explored in concert, they can have a powerfully catalyzing effect on the process of meditation. The following exercises may help you further explore and embody these basic principles.

～ Upright Spine

Whenever you sit down to meditate, spend at least the first few minutes tending to the upright spine. To create an upright spine, the major segments of the torso, like a child's tower of building blocks, need to enter into a balanced relationship with each other, each one resting directly on top of the one underneath it.

However, you can't force these segments to line up, like a soldier responding to a call for attention. You can only feel into them and—always moving in the direction of the least amount of effort and the most amount of buoyancy—let them keep making their own spontaneous adjustments toward the upright. Like homing pigeons drawn back to their nest, our bodies instinctually seek to find greater balance and equilibrium if they're allowed to.

- Sit down on your meditation seat—be it cushion, bench, or chair—and start turning your attention to the major segments of the torso that rest above the supporting base of your pelvis and legs: your belly and lower back, your chest and upper back, your shoulder girdle, your neck, your head. One by one, let yourself start feeling into all these segments with the help of your breath.
- Begin by imagining that your inhaled breath doesn't just stop at the lungs, but continues right down into your pelvis and legs. Breathe all the way down, into your pelvis, into and through your legs, and let yourself feel whatever sensations you find there. The pelvis and legs form the base of support for the upright spine, and the sacrum at the back of the pelvis is where the spine begins. As you breathe into your pelvis and legs, feel how breath and awareness can bring sensations alive.
- Move your awareness upward, and take a number of breaths from the diaphragm down into your belly, lower spine, and pelvic bowl, paying special attention to the sensations you feel in the lumbar vertebrae of your spine. Fill your entire belly with the breath, and find where it can be felt to rest the most effortlessly above the supporting base of the pelvis and legs.
- Keep moving upward, and take several breaths into your upper torso, from the diaphragm up to the base of the

neck, feeling breath spreading through your chest and upper back, paying special attention to the sensations, energies, and motions you can feel in your thoracic spine. Let the feeling presence of your upper torso find its way to balance, directly above the belly and the pelvis.

- ◆ Move your awareness to your shoulder girdle, which rests like an oxen's yoke on your spine and rib cage. Feel your shoulder girdle, your arms, and your hands letting go as you breathe, so they too can join in the play of balance.

- ◆ Now feel your neck—the fleshy part of your neck as well as the sensations in each vertebra of the cervical spine. As you breathe in and out, imagine that your breath activates every single sensation in every single cell of your neck.

- ◆ And finally, feel your head, the uppermost segment of your body—its fleshy coverings, the bony cranium, the brain and brain stem and everything they attach to. Feel how your head can balance itself—through the connecting, and very pliable, link of the neck—on top of everything underneath it, like a crown resting on top of a prince's head.

Like a child building a snowman, feel how all these segments want to stack up in a way that supports them all. In reality, you can't ever separate these segments of the spine and the body into discrete, individual components like the rolled balls of snow that form the lower body, torso, and head of a snowman. From the sacrum through the lumbar, thoracic, and cervical vertebrae, through the brain stem and the brain, the spine is all one interconnected piece. Once you're able to feel sensations in each individual segment, you can start broadening your focus so you can feel the entire spine all at once, from coccyx to cranium, as an integrated system, filled with vibratory sensation, as potentially fluid in its play of verticality as a seahorse in the ocean.

When you sit down to mediate, don't be in too much of a hurry to start focusing on your breath. Pay attention, as the Buddha suggests, to the upright spine first. And keep coming back to it, from time to time, throughout your practice. Its shape and sensations are constantly changing, breath by breath. Playing with balance creates a more watery environment in which the upright spine can be felt to float and through which the breath can be felt to pass. At times you may even want to turn your meditation practice solely into an exploration of the upright, floating, liberated spine.

～ Upside-Down Broom

Can you remember a time as a child when you played with a broom, balancing it upside down on your hand, so the tip of the shaft was resting on your palm and the fibers of the broom were floating high above your head? Few things more effectively demonstrate how gravity supports objects whose structures are predominantly vertical. While it looks to a young mind as though magic is at work, the upside-down broom, hovering effortlessly in the air, is just obeying the laws of physics.

- When you sit in meditation, imagine that your spine is like the broom, balancing itself as effortlessly as possible above the supporting base of your pelvis and legs.

~ The Moving Spine

Upright balance is never a static state. It can only be entered into as a play of movement that never stops. The upright spine isn't like a monolithic, architectural column from a Greek or Roman temple. It's composed not of one solid piece, but of twenty-four individual vertebral bones plus the fused segments of the sacrum and coccyx. The joints between the individual vertebrae of the spine are not unlike joints anywhere else in the body. They exist solely for the purpose of movement.

The spine is designed to move in a natural, undulating motion as we breathe, but we don't normally allow this motion to occur or appreciate its value. We settle instead into restrictive patterns of holding that keep portions of our spine still and unmoving. The play of balance that tends to the upright spine begins by feeling sensations line up congruently, as though they were self-organizing around the vertical. It continues through letting movement course through the body as we breathe in and out.

◆ Sometimes, as you sit in meditation, turn your attention to your spine, and start allowing movement to occur between each and every vertebra in response to the breath. On every inhalation, feel each vertebra move as part of a larger coordinated wave flowing through a lengthening spine. On every exhalation, notice how the spine settles back down. Keep moving your awareness through your spine, vertebra by vertebra. How does each one want to move on the breath, to shift its angle and the distance between itself and its adjacent neighbor? What happens when you forget to let it move? Once the vertebrae start moving on the breath, movement starts spreading more easily through the joints of the rest of the body.

Exploring upright balance in your sitting posture is like riding a bicycle, not like positioning a fence post. If you're frozen and stiff, you'll keep falling off the bike, but if you stay loose and flexible, constantly letting the body make its spontaneous adjustments to balance, you will glide down the road.

～ Befriending Stillness

Ordinarily, we hide the places in our body that don't move from ourselves. They're often painful, and they may even be repositories for shadowy energies and parts of ourselves that we don't really want to have much to do with. Life only knows movement, so if there are things in our life we'd rather not feel—our sadnesses, our fears, even our hopes that we somehow have been led to believe are unrealistic—we can dissociate ourselves from them by locking them away inside secret chests of stillness. As we keep opening to the possibility that subtle motion can be felt to occur between the vertebrae as a natural response to the breath, we inevitably discover areas in our spine that don't seem to move very much at all as we breathe.

Maybe it's your head and neck that don't move much. Maybe it's your chest, your upper back, your shoulders. Maybe it's your arms that never move, never ride the waves of the breath, as you breathe in and out. Maybe it's your belly, your lower back, your diaphragm. Holding still in any of these areas of the body will freeze the vertebrae in that area. Only after you've located where you brace yourself against the natural motions that the breath wants to make can you start to let go.

Then, slowly and gently over time, restrictions to breath can start releasing and coming undone.

◆ As you sit in meditation, ask yourself the following questions:

> *Where do I feel the most movement in my spine in*
> *response to the breath?*
> *Where do I feel the least?*
> *Where do I hold myself still?*
> *What parts of my body don't move when I breathe?*

Never shun or create aversion toward the still places in your body. Don't avoid or try to jump over them as though they're just inconveniences along the way. We all have a unique way in which we hold back and inhibit the breath. Only by bringing the sensations of stillness and holding to awareness is the possibility for movement reborn. Befriend the still places in your spine. See if you can determine their location as precisely as possible. The still places in your body, once located and felt into, hold the key to their own resolution back into movement.

〜 Feeling Presence

Always remember to let yourself feel the body. The activity in every little cell of the body generates tiny pinpricks of rapidly changing sensation whose vibratory nature can be felt throughout the entire body as flow and shimmer. To familiarize yourself with the extraordinary range, colorings, and textures of the body's sensations, it is helpful to start by slowly moving your awareness through each and every part of the body, leaving nothing out.

◆ Begin by turning your attention to the very top of the head. Focus your awareness on an area no bigger than a large coin, just at the top of the head, and let yourself feel whatever sensations can be felt in this one small part of the body. The varieties of sensation you can encounter are endless, and their different colorings and shadings are far more numerous than the words we have to describe them (tingling, vibrating, aching, light, cool, heavy, pulsing, painful, dull, crisp, ecstatic, warm . . .). So don't be overly concerned about whether you can name sensations; just let yourself feel them.

◆ Once you're able to feel a distinct sensation of one kind or another at the top of your head, start broadening your focus to include the adjacent parts of the body. Spread your awareness slowly, an eighth of an inch at a time, and feel what your entire scalp area feels like, what your ears feel like, your forehead, your temples. Feel your eyes and nose, your cheekbones, your mouth, tongue, and teeth. Feel the sensations at the surface of your face as well as the sensations in the center of your cranium. Let yourself feel your entire head—its individual parts as well as the head as a whole. Don't be in a hurry.

◆ In the beginning it may be easier to feel sensations out at the surface of the body, but over time, as your awareness becomes sharper, you'll be able to feel sensations deep in the interior of the body as well. Place your attention on the sensations at the front of your face, and then slowly pass your feeling awareness right through your cranium until you come to the back of your head. Similarly, you can turn your attention to one side of your head and then pass your awareness through to the other side.

• Inch by inch, the texture and feeling tone of sensations can completely change. Don't ever try to force sensations to feel like anything other than they are—vibrating, compacted, spacious, condensed, numb, blissful, or deeply painful. Just by feeling them, exactly as they are, they start changing on their own, releasing, letting go, shifting, intensifying, shimmering, relaxing your held tensions.

• Move your awareness down into your neck. Feel the sensations in the front of your throat, the back and sides of your neck, tiny wavelets of sensations flickering on and off, changing tone and texture from one micro-moment to the next. Once you've been able to register sensations on the surface areas of the neck, pass your attention from the front of your throat right through to the back of your neck. Start on one side of the neck, and pass your attention through the interior mass of the neck out to the surface of the other side.

• Feel your shoulders and your arms. Can you relax your shoulders and arms so they just hang, naturally, off the sides of your torso? Follow the sensations down your arms into the palms and backs of your hands and into each of your fingers. The palms of the hands are especially fertile ground for sensations. If you're having trouble understanding what sensation is, it can be helpful to stay focused on feeling the open, upturned palms of your hands for some time.

• Turn your attention to your upper torso—your chest, the sides of your rib cage, your entire upper back area. If you come across shimmer and vibration, watch these sensations continue to flow. If you come across areas of pain or tension, see if you can relax them. Just to the left of center, in the mid-

dle of your chest, the heart beats like a drum. Can you feel
the beating of your heart?

- Turn your attention to your belly, lower back, and the con-
tents of the entire bowl of the pelvis. Starting at the front of
the belly, slowly pass your awareness right into and through
the body, so that you come out in the back, feeling everything you can along the way. Pass your awareness from side to
side.

- And finally, let yourself feel the sensations in your legs—your
upper legs, your knees, your lower legs and ankles, your feet
and toes.

- Never attempt to manipulate or create sensations. Just feel
what's there to be felt exactly as it is. As you place attention
on a part of the body, opening to whatever can be felt to exist
there, sensations will start appearing and changing on their
own. According to one of the most intriguing principles of
modern physics, whenever you observe an object or event,
you affect and alter the object or event being observed. Turning your attention to your body brings its sensational presence to life.

We are all, to a greater or lesser degree, subject to the
somatophobic bias of our culture, which overvalues the work-
ings of the mind while denigrating the experience of the body
and ends up creating a tragic schism between the two. But this
conditioning can be reversed. As you keep passing your awareness through your body, over and over again, more and more
sensations naturally start appearing, like stars above the desert
that come out one by one in the early evening, only to fill the
entire sky by midnight.

As you explore the possibilities of breathing through the whole body, you may want to alternate between periods in which you feel the entire body all at once, as a unified presence, and times when you move your awareness much more slowly through each and every part of the body in sequence. When you can feel the whole body all at once, it becomes easier for a breath to move through its entire mass. When the mind starts wandering and the feeling presence of the body becomes too diffuse, then shift your focus back to moving your awareness part by part again, through the whole body, over and over, resurrecting the body once again, sensation by sensation.

Merging the awareness of the feeling presence of the body with the natural motions of breath ushers you very directly into the territory of breathing through the whole body. In some of the body-oriented forms of Theravadin Buddhism that are practiced in southeast Asia, passing awareness through the sensations of the entire body, over and over again, forms a stand-alone centerpiece of an extremely potent path of practice.

～ Drawing Down

Ordinarily, we think of an inhalation as raising us up, as extending the spine and head upward. However, to breathe through the whole body, to allow all the movements that naturally want to occur, you don't in any way want to artificially create or encourage upward extension, such as a model walking down a runway or a soldier standing at attention might. You will want instead to surrender the weight of the body to gravity as though a stone were falling through the body, dropping way down deep into the interior of the earth. Newton suggested that for every action taken, an equal and opposite reaction naturally occurs. Dropping slightly down at the onset of an inhalation generates a natural upward lifting by the end of the inhalation.

- Sitting in meditation, playing with upright balance, start surrendering as much of the weight of your body as you can to the pull of gravity without collapsing in any way. From the top of your head down through the tip of your sacrum, right through the core of your body, just feel the weight of your body dropping and letting go, as though it were water draining off your body in a shower, and time this gesture of relaxation to coincide with the sudden onset of inhalation. Dropping suddenly down in this way helps free up the physical holdings and restrictions that constrain and inhibit breath, and breath invariably becomes deeper and fuller. As it deepens in this way, it can be felt to pass through, influence, touch, and include more of the body.

The most important piece of the practice of *Drawing Down* is the initiatory dropping of the weight at the beginning of the inhalation. By relaxing the body and surrendering its weight to the pull of gravity, breath has no choice but to be drawn down into the lungs on the inhalation, like iron filings being pulled toward a magnetic source. And then, as the breath turns and the exhalation begins, the air can just as naturally be felt to rush back up, through, and out of the body. This down and up motion of the breath—drawing down on the inhalation, passing back up and out on the exhalation—can be felt as alternating waves of sensation, as the rush of air races down into the body, turns right around and races back up and out.

～ *The Breath of the Unfolding Fern*

In the forests and gardens of coastal British Columbia where I've lived for the past thirty years, one of the first signs of spring's return is the appearance of tiny, new fern fronds emerging out of the earth. The root stalk is strong and sturdy, but the upper end of the fern is much more delicate and coils down protectively on itself like the top half of a wound-up question mark. As the fern grows and matures, the coils unwind until the frond reaches its full, extended adult length. The life cycle of a fern frond begins by uncoiling itself in the spring and ends by dropping away over the winter. The life cycle of an individual breath goes through the same phases of growth and decay and can even be felt to mimic the frond's motions.

- As you sit in meditation, let your head come slightly forward at the end of an exhalation. Drop and angle your forehead a bit down toward the floor, but not so far down that you come anywhere near touching your chin to your chest. As you incline your head slightly forward and down, your gaze will momentarily rest on a spot on the floor a few feet in front of you. This is the position of the young, uncoiled fern, wound down naturally on itself. And this is where the new cycle of breath is born again.

- Begin by suddenly dropping the weight of your body down into the earth, and coordinate this gesture of relaxation with the onset of your inhalation. The motions of breath rush down from the diaphragm into the belly, lower back, and pelvis, while rushing upward through the torso, neck, and head. As the force of the breath reaches your bowed head, it creates a hydraulic pressure, a natural pumping motion, and the cervical spine starts uncoiling itself backward and upward until, at the height of the inhalation, the head has been lifted up by the breath and your gaze is more directly in front of you.

- The cycle of the breath turns. On the exhalation, everything starts collapsing down on itself again. The head drops forward and back down as the cervical spine recoils. It's as though the fern frond opens out through its entire length on the inhalation and falls back into its original coiled state on the exhalation.

- While motion can be felt throughout the entire spine, the most prominent motion occurs in the head and neck. Viewed from the side, the chin traces a circular path, over and over again. At the onset of inhalation, the chin drops slightly and then starts moving backward as though it's tucking itself into the neck. Then it rises up in conjunction with the filling of the lungs. And finally, it moves forward and drops back down on the exhalation. Breath after breath, it repeats this natural, circular motion.

It is helpful to explore *The Breath of the Unfolding Fern* as a conscious exercise if you ever start feeling groggy or lost in your practice, as it invariably points you back in the direction of breathing through your whole body. Coordinate the timing of the top of your inhalation with the full uncoiling of the spine. Coordinate the very bottom of the exhalation with the recoiling of the spine and the slight dropping down and forward of the head. In this way, the body stays in constant motion—uncoiling on the inhalation, recoiling on the exhalation, rocking on the pelvis. Make sure the entire spine moves in one fluid motion as you breathe in and out.

The primal impulse to breathe comes from the very center of the body and the very core of being. So, the movements and perpetual motion of the breath must emerge from the inside out, not be imposed from the outside in. Are you overly participating in the action of breath, controlling its patterns of inhalation and exhalation, or are you just surrendering to it, yielding to its primal power, letting go as best you can of whatever obstructions to its motion you discover? From one breath to the next, just keep letting breath breathe you however it wants.

～ Rocking the Pelvis

While the head balances on the very top of the spine, the pelvis forms the supporting base at the very bottom of the spine. Just as the head can remain in constant, circular motion as you breathe in and out, so too can the pelvis keep rocking back and forth on every inhalation and exhalation. In a highly frozen sitting posture, however, the pelvis mostly remains as unmoving as the head. To experience a breath that breathes through the whole body, movement needs to be invited back into the pelvis every bit as much as it needs to occur in the head.

◆ As you sit in meditation, let your pelvis start rocking back and forth over the fulcrum of your sitting bones, and coordinate this movement with the inhalation and exhalation of breath. As you inhale, rock your hips forward over your pelvis. As you do this, the lumbar spine will naturally thrust itself forward as well. This strong, pronounced motion in the pelvis and lumbar spine gets immediately transferred up the whole length of the spine, and the head has no choice but to bob upward and slightly back in response.

- On the exhalation, the motions reverse themselves. The pelvis rocks backward over the sitting bones. The lumbar spine curves backward as well, and as it does, the head naturally drops forward and down.
- Through this rocking motion at the pelvis, the entire spine—from the sacrum up through the brain stem—remains in constant, fluid motion. No holding anywhere. No stillness anywhere. Just constant movement throughout the spine, movement that never ever stops.
- At the beginning, let the rocking movement back and forth at the pelvis be quite pronounced. At first this may feel strange, especially in the context of what we ordinarily consider to be the largely nonmoving quality of the meditation posture. After ten or fifteen minutes, however, this pumping motion of the rocking pelvis will start feeling much more natural. If you now bring the movement to a forced stoppage, the frozen stillness that returns—common as it may be to so many sitting meditators—starts feeling decidedly uncomfortable and unnatural. So let the pelvis go again. Let it start rocking on the breath, forward and back. Let the rest of the spine respond and participate, constantly moving, never coming to rest.
- At times, especially if you're feeling sluggish and out of touch with body and breath, you can exaggerate this movement so that, on the inhalation, the spine becomes markedly lengthened and uncoiled while, on the exhalation, the spine becomes highly compressed and rounded. As body and breath come back to life, and as mind starts clearing and settling down, the rocking movement will naturally become less pronounced, but it never ever disappears or comes to a standstill.

As you sit on your cushion, keep exploring *Rocking the Pelvis* and *The Breath of the Unfolding Fern* as two parts of the same, coordinated exercise. In this way, the spine stays in constant, resilient motion, body lets go of unnecessary tension and holding, and mind has no solid foundation on which to build a litany of unbidden thoughts.

～ Floating Shoulders, Sinking Hands

Much like the long, horizontal bar that a tightrope walker carries as he moves across a taut cable tied between two buildings, arms and shoulders function as lateral supports that help stabilize upright balance. A tightrope walker makes constant, small adjustments to the angle and positioning of the bar, and the subtle shifting of weight that occurs helps keep him glued to the wire under his feet.

A meditator who sits with an unmoving head and neck will almost certainly freeze her arms and shoulders as well. Just as the tightrope walker's bar stays in motion to keep him balanced, so can the shoulders, arms, and hands of a meditator resiliently ride on the breath, like driftwood riding up and down ocean swells.

* Whether you rest your hands on your knees or fold them in your lap, your elbows will hang at around the level of your lower rib cage, not far from where the diaphragm separates your upper and lower torsos. In *The Breath of the Unfolding Fern,* everything above the diaphragm uncoils upward on the inhalation while everything below the diaphragm relaxes and settles down. The same can be true of the motions of your arms and shoulders. As you sit in meditation, feel

your lower arms, hands, and fingers relaxing and dropping down on the inhalation. And feel your upper arms, scapulae, and clavicles being lifted ever so slightly up and back to accommodate the volume of air that's rushing in to fill the lungs.

- On the exhalation, the shoulders and upper arms reverse their motions, fall forward and down again, back to where they started, only to begin rising back up on the very next inhalation. The lower arms and hands just keep dropping their weight to the pull of gravity, moving ever so slightly in response to the major motions at the shoulders.

- It is not possible to initiate this rhythmic, repetitive movement in the arms and shoulders and keep the head and neck still and unmoving. As soon as the shoulders start lifting, the neck and head have to start moving in response as well. Don't lift up with your shoulders or chest on the inhalation. Just let them float up, naturally, on the hydraulic pumping action of the breath.

～ Breathing the Six Directions

Upright but deeply relaxed, the whole body can expand and contract, riding on the tidal flow of the breath, constantly moving. The retraction on the exhalation always brings us back toward our center while the expansion on the inhalation moves us outward through the six primary directions: front, back, up, down, left, right. Sometimes, in a deeply relaxed condition, all we need to do is remind ourselves that breath wants to move through the body in all six directions. On every inhalation the torso can be felt to expand both forward and back, the body lengthens both up toward the sky and down into the earth, the right and left sides of the body billow outward, away from each other, like a balloon being blown in to. As we breathe out, everything retracts back in to the center, like a balloon deflating from all directions.

• You may want to familiarize yourself with the possibilities of this most natural of full-bodied breaths by first focusing on individual segments of the torso and exploring the possibility for expansion in the six directions in each of the segments separately.

• Turn your attention first to the belly. Many contemporary Buddhist schools continue to follow the initial instructions in the *Satipatthana Sutta* by having students focus all their attention on how the front wall of the belly can be felt, ever so slightly, to rise on the inhalation and fall back in and down on the exhalation. For this exercise, broaden the possibility of movement that can be felt in the belly to include expansion and contraction not just at the front belly wall, but in all six directions. On the inhalation the belly expands forward, but the lumbar spine can equally be felt to billow out backward. The abdomen lengthens upward but can also be felt to expand downward. The sides of the lower torso swell and reach out, and everything happens all at once. On the exhalation, it's as though the air rushes out of the balloon, and everything retracts back in.

• After a number of conscious breaths, move your attention up to your rib cage. With every inhalation the chest can be felt to expand, increasing its size in all directions, as the inhalation fills the lungs. Each rib can move interdependently in a coordinated, fluid motion. The front of your chest can be felt to expand outward while your spine can be felt, simultaneously, to move backward. The right and left sides of the rib cage can be felt moving away from each other, rocking the shoulders and arms as they do. The entire chest can be felt to lengthen. And then the cycle turns again: the air rushes out, and the chest settles back in.

- Finally, turn your attention to your head and neck and see that these segments of the body, so ordinarily overlooked in the physiology of breathing, can also be felt, in a deeply relaxed body, to expand and contract, ever so slightly, in all six directions, on every inhalation and exhalation.

- Now, put these segments back together into the unified whole that they are, and add your awareness of the meditational base of support on which they all rest—the pelvis, legs, and feet. The whole body, all one unit, can be felt to expand simultaneously up toward the sky, down into the earth, out toward the visual field in front of the body, into the mystery space of feeling presence in the back of the body, out to both the right and the left.

One of the most valuable features of this exercise is that it allows you to pinpoint precisely where in your body you hold yourself still and brace against the force of the breath. The still places in the body function as repositories not only of physical tension, but of the unconscious impulses of the mind as well. Only after you become fully conscious of the feeling quality of resistance and holding can the process of surrendered letting go begin, so as you continue to let go and more movement can be felt returning through the three directional axes—front/back, up/down, right/left—watch how both body and mind are affected. The mind that monologues can only take root in a soil of stillness. Take away the stillness, and what happens to the mind now? What happens to the body? What happens to *you*?

Remember: Breathing through the whole body is not some kind of calisthenic exercise; it is a koan to guide you as you sit down to meditate, a seed possibility that gradually takes root, grows, and matures over time. It is an invitation to include more and more of the feeling presence of the body and to let go of the roadblocks to the free passage of the breath. The exercises can help get you started on your way, but the practice ripens not through repeating a set pattern of steps but through continually yielding to the impulse behind the next breath you're about to take.

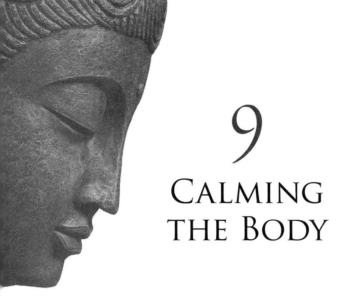

9

CALMING
THE BODY

---

feel how the breath calms and heals* the body

We all have a contraction at the core of our being, right in the center of our body and mind. This contraction makes us who we are, but it also limits us from becoming all that we are. And it hurts. Like a tightened fist, it keeps the life force that wants to pass freely through our body and mind held back and restrained. Its primary tendencies are to compress the energy of the body, like a black hole drawing everything toward its center, and to tether the activity of the mind to the dimension

---

*I've taken a small liberty with the translation of the text by suggesting that breath *heals* as well as calms the body, even though it doesn't appear in any of the accepted translations, because I believe its addition helps clarify the intentions of the text.

of thought. Every time we tense the body in reaction, we add to the contraction, like a beaver adding another twig to a dam. Every moment we relax, the contraction comes undone a bit.

Tension and stillness in the body feed the contraction, and its appetite is large. In whatever shape or pattern it appears in you (we all have unique ways in which we hold tension in our body), the contraction can always be felt to interfere with the free flow of breath. Built of residual patterns of tension and holding, it is the confining force behind the still places in your body that don't move as you breathe.

Exploring the koan of breathing through the whole body in the context of sitting meditation helps soften the contraction. Gradually, breath by surrendered breath, it can start releasing its hold, loosening its grip, revealing, at the level of both body and mind, what it has been holding back all this time. Breath by breath, places in the body with little sensation start coming back to life. Breath by breath, areas of the body that don't move start moving again. Breath by breath, tensions in the body start relaxing. A muscle in chronic tension keeps firing unending signals of contraction in very rapid frequencies. As the tension relaxes and releases, the body becomes calmer, less agitated.

Calming the body of its tensions helps heal the body of its pain. As breath starts breathing through more and more of the body, it becomes a direct agent of healing, massaging and helping to melt any areas of tension it touches into and moves through. In the same way that a bodyworker's hands are able to touch you from the outside in, a breath that keeps the body in unending motion massages you from the inside out, breath by breath, stroke by stroke. You can feel it working on you internally, probing into areas and recesses of tissues that the bodyworker can't put her hands on. Everywhere the breath penetrates, every place it touches and presses into, it activates sensations and promotes the release of tension. Like a current in a river, confronting a logjam, the force of breath pushes up against tension's walls in hopes of dissolving its barriers, turning tension in the body back into shimmer, and contraction in the mind back into presence.

The open dimension of being (*sunyata*) that Mahayana Buddhism promotes as such an important value is the polar opposite of the closed fist of the contraction. For body and mind to open, the tendency to contract needs to be offset by a gesture of letting go, releasing whatever you're holding so tightly to yourself, transforming imploding compression into a relaxation that keeps radiating outward. Exploring the possibilities of a breath that can be felt to breathe through the whole body lets you start opening up, coming out of your held shell, emerging from the shadows cast by contraction's mass.

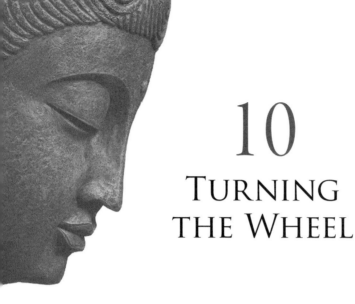

10
TURNING
THE WHEEL

like a skilled potter watching clay turn on a wheel
notice how each inhalation turns into an exhalation
only to turn back again into an inhalation
*over and over and over again**

"Turning the wheel" is a Buddhist term referring to a progressive deepening of the teachings as expressed in a series of discourses the Buddha gave during his life. The wheel of *dharma* (the teachings of the Buddha) was first set into motion through

---

*I've taken some liberties with this verse translation as well. The sutta doesn't specify pottery as the trade, only that it is a trade involving "turning." This could as easily apply to wood or metal work crafted on a lathe, but I've chosen here to focus on pottery. The second part of this verse is a simplification and summation of some of the statements about breath that appeared earlier in the sutta and are repeated again following the image of the potter.

an early discourse about suffering, its causes, and its resolutions. A later turning emphasized the empty and utterly spacious quality of phenomena (we look at other people and see their bodies as being very solid, but when we go inside and feel our own, all we come up with is a feeling presence of empty space and vibratory sensation) as well as the fundamentally compassionate nature of mind. Later turnings would elaborate on the first two, and in this way the full spectrum of Buddhist teachings could be addressed and expanded on. While some Buddhist schools embrace all the successive turnings of the wheel as elaborations and clarifications of the dharma, others focus their practices more exclusively on one of the turnings over the others.

The "turning wheel" referred to in this sutta is a different kind of wheel. It refers not to the deepening of teachings expressed by the Buddha, but to the deepening of understanding that arises for a meditator who keeps his or her attention fixed on the never-ending cycle of breath in which inhalations and exhalations keep turning into each other, over and over and over again.

When it comes to breathing practice, we're not all that different from a potter. Once we sit the clay of our bodies down onto the cushion, we set the wheel of breath in motion and start paying close attention to it, round after round. Like the potter, we have to train ourselves to stay focused and not let the mind wander off. In the same way that the potter learns to understand the secrets of the clay through every turning of the wheel, we become ever more adept at breathing through the whole body every time we open to its possibility.

One of clay's secrets is that you can't just do anything you want with it. It doesn't magically submit to your fingers in the way you'd like to think it should. You have to learn how to work with it and how to listen to it. It has its own stories to tell before it lets you unlock its shapes and forms. Sometimes there may be snags in the clay's story that disrupt the flowing motion of the wheel. The master potter learns how to coax the secrets out of the clay.

A meditator works with body, breath, and mind in much the same way as a potter works with clay, motion, and intention. Sitting in meditation, you settle into your body and start watching your breath, turning, turning. If the potter loses his focus, the clay can fly off the wheel. If you lose your focus, you'll likely spin off into thought. A master potter in a master moment doesn't impose will on the clay, but lets the pot emerge out of it, in its own time, at its own pace, in its own way. The restrictive holding patterns in the body and mind unravel their secrets the same way the potter frees the pot from the clay—through accepting, feeling into, allowing, coaxing, never by forcing.

Breath rarely liberates itself in a straight line or along a two-dimensional plane. Far more common are twists and turns, logjams and releases, a journey of spiral unwindings through the body. What matters more than how you breathe (in and out through the nose, in through the nose and out through the mouth, in and out of the nose and mouth together, etc.) is how you keep surrendering to breath and to the puzzling possibility that it might breathe through more and more of your body. Sometimes the breath can slow down and lengthen; at other times it can speed up in short bursts. Sometimes it may

fade so far away that you can barely feel it; at other times it can explode open, like a steam locomotive racing down a track of rails.

While breathing through the whole body implies that the entire body is constantly, subtly moving, there can be times when everything seems to come to a stop and freezes. At those times it is important to remember that the practice is to surrender to the breath as it learns to make its way through the whole body, never to force it. Sometimes deep sensations and feelings are hidden inside these extended, frozen pauses, waiting to be stirred, unearthed, released. At other times pauses come with a direct invitation to drop down deeper into the silent well in your center. Smooth or choppy, the current of breath keeps flowing, and its cycles keep turning, turning.

Breath is just the means. The real goal of the practice is to experience what happens to you—your mind, your sense of self, your understanding of incarnation—when you explore the possibility of breathing through your whole body. The purpose of Buddhist practices isn't to perfect breath. It's to find out who you are and who you become when you pay attention to it. Ordinarily, our minds rule the roost, and our breath and body stumble along behind, like children trying to catch up to an impatient parent. How different it would be if we gave our breath and body precedence and let our mind align itself with them. And how different still if we could integrate all three elements—mind, body, breath—into a coordinated merging so that they would function in concert as a more unified phenomenon. It would be like lining up the three numbers on a padlock so that it can slide open.

Meditation is for those of us who realize that we've forgotten who we are and would like to remember. Re-membering is literally a process of putting back together again the fractured and scattered pieces that have come apart. Integrating body, mind, and breath through the practice of breathing through the whole body helps us remember.

About the Author

Will Johnson, the author of several books, including *The Posture of Meditation, Yoga of the Mahamudra, Rumi's Four Essential Practices, The Sailfish and the Sacred Mountain,* and the award-winning *The Spiritual Practices of Rumi,* is the founder and director of the Institute for Embodiment Training in British Columbia, Canada. He received his B.A., magna cum laude, in Art and Archaeology from Princeton University in 1968. After working for several years as an art critic in New York, he moved to the west coast of North America and began exploring the practices that would come to be known as Gazing at the Beloved and Sudaba. He became a Buddhist practitioner in 1968, was trained as a Rolfer in 1976, and began the formal sharing of the practices of Embodiment Training in 1995.

For more information, or to receive announcements about programs and retreats based on the principles in this book, please visit the author's website

www.embodiment.net

INDEX

Page numbers followed by "n" indicate notes.